Calm Pregnancy

How I Overcame Anxiety, Stress, and Depression During Pregnancy

Based on True Life Experience

PUBLISHED BY: Bonaventure Consults

Bonaventure Consults

Copyright © 2024. All rights reserved.

No part of this publication may be copied, reproduced in any format, by any means, electronic or otherwise without prior consent from the copyright owner and publisher of this book.

Table of content

Table of content 3

Introduction 4

Chapter 1: My Pregnancy Journey 6

Chapter 2: Understanding Anxiety During Pregnancy 9

Chapter 4: The Prevalence of Anxiety and How It Affects Mothers 25

Chapter 5: How I Overcame Anxiety: Treatment Options That Worked for Me 33

Chapter 6: Practical Techniques for Managing Anxiety in Pregnancy 40

Chapter 7: How Anxiety Affects Your Baby and What You Can Do About It 48

Chapter 8: Managing Fear of Labor and Delivery (Tokophobia) 55

Chapter 9: Finding Your Calm: Daily Habits for Long-Term Peace 63

Conclusion 71

About the Author 75

Disclaimer 76

Acknowledgement 77

Introduction

Sitting on a cozy armchair on my balcony, the fresh ocean breeze washing over me, I watched the waves roll in and felt the weight of my baby daughter in my arms. She had just turned one, a bright and beautiful soul, and here I was, a tear sliding down my cheek. The journey to this moment had been nothing short of miraculous.

As I rocked her gently, I couldn't help but reflect on the whirlwind of emotions I'd experienced during pregnancy—especially the fear, anxiety, and depression that nearly consumed me. I had walked through fire and come out stronger. Anxiety and depression during pregnancy are real, and they affect countless women. But they aren't the end of the story. With the right support and a few simple techniques, I found my way out. And so can you.

In this book, I share my personal journey, how I overcame anxiety and postpartum depression, and the practical steps I took to regain control of my mental health. It's not just my story; it's a guide that includes practical, easy-to-follow tips for every expectant mother feeling overwhelmed by anxiety or stress. This book is meant to be both a comforting friend and a roadmap for navigating the emotional roller coaster that pregnancy can often be.

Together, we'll explore the techniques that helped me, the proven strategies from professionals, and the best ways to prepare mentally and emotionally for the incredible task of bringing new life into the world.

Chapter 1: My Pregnancy Journey

My pregnancy journey was not an easy road. It was filled with heartache, uncertainty, and emotional highs and lows that I never anticipated. I had been married for over ten years to my childhood sweetheart, a man who stood by me through thick and thin. Our love story was beautiful, but it wasn't without its share of challenges. After nine years of waiting, I experienced my second miscarriage. The emotional toll was unbearable. I felt shattered, lost, and utterly defeated. To make things worse, my husband had recently lost his job, adding financial stress to an already fragile emotional state.

The feelings of failure, both as a wife and as a future mother, overwhelmed me. I felt broken and helpless, unable to understand why things were falling apart when all I wanted was a family. My mental state began to spiral out of control. I turned to comfort eating, indulging in junk food, as if it could somehow fill the emotional void. But food could never heal the deep wounds I was carrying.

It was at this point that I made a deliberate decision—I had to seek help, not just from others but from within myself. It was a realization that only I could take the first step to recovery. With my husband's constant support and encouragement, I began my journey of self-help. Slowly, I started to pull myself back from the edge.

That same year, as if by miracle, I conceived again. But rather than pure joy, I felt a confusing mix of emotions—fear, anxiety, and disbelief. I wasn't ready for another pregnancy. My mind had not healed from the previous losses. I was caught between the urge to terminate the pregnancy and the hope that this time, things would be different. After much thought and consultation with my family and a trusted counselor, I decided to fight for this pregnancy.

I won't lie—my first trimester was nothing short of a nightmare. Constantly plagued by flashbacks of my miscarriages, I was overwhelmed with nausea, heartburn, and an utter inability to sleep. Each night, my mind filled with worst-case scenarios: What if I lost this baby too? What if I wasn't strong enough? What if something terrible happened?

These thoughts led to frequent panic attacks, where I would find myself unable to breathe, my heart racing, and my body shaking uncontrollably. The feeling of dread was suffocating, and it made every aspect of my life seem impossible. The anxiety consumed me.

But this time, unlike before, I knew I needed to address these emotions head-on. I couldn't let fear control me, especially with a new life growing inside me. Through counseling, talking openly with my family, and using specific techniques I'll share later in this book, I began to regain a sense of calm and control. It wasn't easy, and I had many setbacks along the way, but gradually, I found the tools that worked for me.

As the pregnancy progressed, I learned the value of self-compassion, trusting in the process, and leaning on a strong support system. I had to accept that there would be moments of weakness, but those didn't define me as a mother or a woman. Each day brought new lessons, and eventually, those dark clouds of anxiety began to lift. I gave birth to my daughter—a healthy, vibrant, beautiful girl—proving to myself that I could overcome the impossible.

This journey taught me that anxiety in pregnancy is not something to be ashamed of. It's a common struggle that many women face, and with the right approach, it can be managed and even overcome. The techniques I used were simple, but they worked. My hope is that by sharing my story and these strategies, other women will feel empowered to face their own struggles with anxiety, knowing they are not alone.

Chapter 2: Understanding Anxiety During Pregnancy

Pregnancy is often portrayed as one of the most joyful and exciting times in a woman's life. But for many of us, it's also a time filled with anxiety, fear, and uncertainty. I remember when I first found out I was pregnant, I expected to be nothing but overjoyed, but instead, I found myself overwhelmed with worry. The truth is, while the joy and anticipation of bringing new life into the world are real, so too are the fears and anxieties that accompany such a life-changing event.

Understanding anxiety during pregnancy was a pivotal moment for me. Before I understood what was happening, I blamed myself for feeling the way I did. I questioned why I wasn't constantly happy, and why I couldn't relax and just enjoy the experience. It wasn't until I began learning about pregnancy-related anxiety that I realized these feelings were not only common, but they were also a completely normal response to the significant physical, emotional, and psychological changes I was going through.

The Source of My Anxiety

For me, pregnancy anxiety started early. From the moment I found out I was expecting, my mind was flooded with questions. Some were practical—about how I would handle the physical demands of pregnancy and whether I was financially prepared. But others were deeper, more existential questions. Would I be a good mother? Could I provide my child with the love, support, and security they needed? Would I be able to handle the labor and delivery process?

At times, these worries felt all-consuming. I noticed that my anxiety intensified when I was alone with my thoughts, especially at night. I would lie in bed, wide awake, replaying all the possible scenarios in my mind. My heart would race, and my body would tense up. It was as though I was bracing myself for something terrible to happen, even though nothing was wrong in that moment.

The anxiety was amplified by hormonal changes that came with pregnancy. I knew that my body was undergoing massive transformations to support the growing life inside of me, but I hadn't anticipated how much my emotional landscape would shift as well. I would go from feeling relatively calm to suddenly being overwhelmed by emotions—whether it was fear, anger, or sadness.

These emotional shifts made me feel even more out of control, and that lack of control only fed my anxiety further.

The Impact of Hormonal Changes on Anxiety

One of the first things I learned about pregnancy-related anxiety is how much of it is tied to the hormonal changes happening in our bodies. Hormones like estrogen and progesterone are crucial for supporting a healthy pregnancy, but they also play a major role in regulating mood. As these hormone levels fluctuate, it's normal to experience changes in mood, energy levels, and emotional responses.

For me, the mood swings were one of the most challenging aspects of pregnancy. One day, I would feel excited and optimistic about the future, and the next day, I would be overwhelmed with fear and worry. These emotional highs and lows left me feeling disoriented and disconnected from myself. I kept wondering if I was losing control or if I would ever feel "normal" again.

I soon realized that these emotional fluctuations weren't a reflection of my ability to handle pregnancy—they were simply my body's way of adjusting to the profound changes happening internally. Once I accepted this, I began to develop more self-compassion. Instead of berating myself for feeling anxious, I started to see it as a natural response to everything I was going through.

The Role of Fear in Pregnancy Anxiety

Fear was at the core of much of my anxiety. I was afraid of so many things, both big and small. Some of my fears were rational, while others were exaggerated by the heightened emotions that come with pregnancy. One of the most persistent fears I had was about my baby's health. I worried constantly about whether my baby was developing properly, whether they would be born healthy, and whether I was doing enough to take care of them.

Even though my doctor reassured me that my pregnancy was progressing normally, the anxiety persisted. I found myself seeking out more information—reading articles online, asking friends and family about their experiences, and constantly monitoring my symptoms. While some of this research helped ease my mind, much of it had the opposite effect. I became hyper-focused on every possible complication, and this only fed my anxiety further.

Another major source of fear was the uncertainty of labor and delivery. I had heard so many stories from other women about how painful, difficult, or even traumatic childbirth could be. The more I thought about it, the more terrified I became. I started to question whether I would be able to handle the pain, whether I would make the right decisions during labor, and whether something might go wrong. This fear of the unknown was one of the hardest aspects of pregnancy anxiety for me to cope with.

Anxiety Around Life Changes

Pregnancy isn't just a physical transformation—it's a major life change that brings with it a whole new set of responsibilities. For me, the realization that I was about to become a mother added a new layer of anxiety. I began questioning my readiness for motherhood. I wondered if I would be able to balance my career and family life, whether I had the emotional capacity to care for a child, and how my relationship with my husband might change once the baby arrived.

I worried about whether I was ready to make the sacrifices that come with parenthood. Would I lose my sense of self? Would I be able to continue pursuing my passions, or would my life be completely consumed by caring for my child? These questions were difficult to answer, and the uncertainty of what was to come often left me feeling overwhelmed.

On top of these personal concerns, I also felt pressure from societal expectations. There's a lot of emphasis on the idea that pregnancy

ful, happy time, and when I didn't feel that way, I ted to question whether I was "doing pregnancy ıer my anxiety somehow meant I wasn't cut out to be a mother. It took me a while to understand that there is no right or wrong way to experience pregnancy—everyone's journey is different, and it's okay to have a range of emotions.

How Anxiety Manifests Physically

One thing that surprised me was how much my anxiety manifested physically. It wasn't just about racing thoughts or feeling emotionally overwhelmed—my body reacted to my anxiety in ways that I hadn't anticipated. I experienced frequent headaches, muscle tension, and digestive issues that I later learned were all linked to stress. There were days when my shoulders and neck felt so tight that I could barely move, and I often had trouble sleeping because my body couldn't seem to relax.

Sleep, in particular, was a struggle for me. I would lie awake for hours, my mind racing with worries about the future. Even when I was exhausted, my body wouldn't cooperate, and I'd spend most of the night tossing and turning. This lack of sleep only compounded my anxiety, as I knew how important rest was for both my health and my baby's development.

I also noticed that my heart would race whenever I felt particularly anxious, and there were times when I felt short of breath or dizzy. These physical symptoms were scary because they made the anxiety feel even more real. It wasn't just something happening in my mind—it was affecting my entire body. Once I started paying attention to these physical cues, I realized how deeply interconnected my mind and body were, and I knew that managing my anxiety would require me to address both.

The Importance of Self-Awareness

Through all of this, one of the most valuable lessons I learned was the importance of self-awareness. Understanding the sources of my anxiety and recognizing how it was affecting me—both mentally and physically—allowed me to take steps to manage it more effectively. It wasn't about eliminating anxiety altogether, but rather about learning to respond to it in healthier ways.

I began to notice patterns in my anxiety—times of day when it was worse, specific triggers that set it off, and physical symptoms that signaled when it was escalating. This awareness helped me feel more in control because it gave me the information I needed to take action before the anxiety spiraled out of control.

Self-awareness also helped me become more compassionate with myself. Instead of blaming myself for feeling anxious, I started to view it as a natural response to the changes I was going through. I realized that it was okay to feel anxious, and that the key was finding ways to manage those feelings rather than suppressing or ignoring them.

Chapter 3: Recognizing the Signs: Anxiety, Panic Attacks, and Stress

Pregnancy brings a wide range of emotions—joy, excitement, anticipation—but for many of us, it also brings anxiety, stress, and even panic. As I progressed through my pregnancy, there were moments when I wasn't sure whether what I was feeling was just normal pregnancy worry or something more intense. I began to realize that it was important to recognize when my feelings had crossed the line into anxiety and panic, and how these emotions were affecting me physically, emotionally, and mentally.

Looking back, I can see that my anxiety during pregnancy manifested in different ways. At first, it was subtle—just a constant hum of worry in the background. But as time went on, it grew louder and more disruptive. The worry wasn't just an occasional thought anymore; it became a daily presence, often overshadowing the excitement I wanted to feel. Recognizing the signs of anxiety was the first step in learning how to manage it, and I'm so grateful I didn't ignore those signals.

The Early Signs of Anxiety

At the beginning of my pregnancy, I didn't immediately recognize that I was experiencing anxiety. I thought my constant worrying was just part of the normal experience of becoming a mother. But over time, the worrying intensified. I found myself unable to relax, even when I tried to focus on positive things. There was always a nagging thought in the back of my mind, reminding me of everything that could go wrong.

For me, anxiety often showed up in the form of constant "what if" thinking. What if something went wrong during the pregnancy? What if I wasn't doing enough to protect my baby? What if I wasn't prepared for motherhood? These thoughts would swirl in my mind, making it difficult to focus on anything else.

I also noticed that my anxiety wasn't just mental—it began to show up physically. I would get headaches, feel nauseous, and have trouble sleeping. My body was telling me that something wasn't right, even when I wasn't fully aware of it. Over time, I learned to recognize these physical symptoms as early signs that my anxiety was getting out of control.

How Anxiety Affected My Daily Life

As my pregnancy progressed, I realized that my anxiety wasn't just a passing feeling—it was starting to affect my daily life. I had trouble concentrating on work and found it difficult to enjoy time with friends and family. Even when I was surrounded by people who loved and supported me, I couldn't shake the feeling that something bad was going to happen.

One of the most frustrating parts of anxiety was how unpredictable it could be. I might have a relatively calm day, only to suddenly be hit with a wave of panic or worry for no apparent reason. This made it hard for me to plan or enjoy anything fully because I never knew when the anxiety would show up.

For example, I remember going to a prenatal appointment feeling relatively calm, only to have a minor comment from the doctor about something routine send me into a spiral of fear. Even though the comment was harmless, my mind immediately latched onto it and turned it into a worst-case scenario. I couldn't stop thinking about it for days, replaying the conversation in my head and worrying that something terrible was about to happen.

Recognizing Panic Attacks

One of the most intense and frightening experiences of anxiety during my pregnancy was my first panic attack. It came out of nowhere—at least, that's what it felt like at the time. I was sitting at home, trying to relax, when suddenly, my heart started racing. I felt like I couldn't breathe, and a wave of fear washed over me so quickly that I couldn't make sense of it. My chest tightened, and I thought I was having a heart attack. My mind was screaming, "Something is wrong!"

I later learned that what I experienced was a panic attack—a sudden and intense surge of fear that triggers physical symptoms like shortness of breath, chest pain, dizziness, and a racing heart. At the time, it was terrifying because I had no idea what was happening. It felt like my body was betraying me.

The worst part about panic attacks was that they seemed to come out of nowhere. Even when I was trying to relax or distract myself, the panic would hit without warning. It was like my body was on high alert all the time, and any small trigger could set it off. After my first panic attack, I became even more anxious, constantly fearing the next one. I would lie in bed at night, waiting for it to happen again, which only made my anxiety worse.

The Connection Between Anxiety and Physical Symptoms

One of the things I didn't expect during pregnancy was how much my anxiety would manifest physically. At first, I thought my headaches, nausea, and muscle tension were just part of the normal pregnancy experience. But as time went on, I started to notice a pattern—these symptoms were worse on days when my anxiety was particularly high.

My heart would race, my breathing would become shallow, and I'd feel dizzy or lightheaded. There were days when I felt like I couldn't catch my breath, even though I knew nothing was physically wrong. I learned that these were physical symptoms of anxiety, my body's way of reacting to the stress my mind was experiencing.

For me, the physical symptoms of anxiety were sometimes more overwhelming than the mental ones. It's one thing to have racing thoughts, but it's another to feel like your body is completely out of your control. Recognizing that these physical sensations were connected to my anxiety helped me realize that I needed to address the underlying stress to start feeling better.

The Role of Stress in My Anxiety

Pregnancy is stressful enough on its own, but for me, there were additional life stresses that made my anxiety worse. I was worried about finances, my job, and how my life would change once the baby arrived. These worries piled on top of the anxiety I already felt about the pregnancy, making everything feel more overwhelming.

There were times when I felt like I was trying to juggle too many things at once. I was constantly thinking about all the things I had to prepare for—the nursery, the birth plan, the baby supplies—and it felt like there wasn't enough time to do it all. This constant pressure to "get everything right" made it hard for me to relax and enjoy the pregnancy. I felt like I was always in problem-solving mode, trying to stay ahead of everything, but instead, I was burning out.

How I Learned to Recognize and Manage Anxiety

Once I began to understand the signs of anxiety and how it was affecting me, I knew I had to find ways to manage it before it got worse. The first step for me was acknowledging that what I was experiencing wasn't something I could just push through or ignore. I needed to address it head-on.

One of the most helpful things I did was start tracking my symptoms. I kept a journal where I wrote down when I felt anxious, what triggered it, and how it affected me physically and mentally. This helped me identify patterns—like how my anxiety was often worse at night or how certain situations, like medical appointments, tended to trigger panic.

Once I recognized these patterns, I started working on strategies to manage the anxiety before it escalated into a panic attack. Breathing exercises were a game-changer for me. I practiced deep belly breathing whenever I felt my heart racing or my thoughts spiraling. By focusing on my breath, I was able to calm my body and slow down the anxiety.

Another strategy that helped was learning to challenge my anxious thoughts. I realized that much of my anxiety was fueled by worst-case scenarios that weren't likely to happen. So, when I noticed my mind going down that path, I'd ask myself, "Is this thought based on fact, or is it my anxiety talking?" This simple question helped me separate my fears from reality.

Seeking Help

There came a point in my pregnancy when I realized that managing anxiety on my own wasn't enough—I needed outside support. Talking to my doctor was a huge relief. I explained what I was going through, and she reassured me that anxiety during pregnancy is common. She also encouraged me to seek therapy, which became a crucial part of my anxiety management.

Through therapy, I learned more about the connection between anxiety and pregnancy and gained tools to manage my anxiety in healthier ways. My therapist helped me work through my fears about labor, motherhood, and the future, giving me a sense of control over my mental health.

If you're experiencing anxiety or panic attacks during pregnancy, know that it's okay to ask for help. Whether it's talking to your doctor, seeing a therapist, or reaching out to a support group, getting the help you need can make a world of difference. You don't have to go through this alone.

Chapter 4: The Prevalence of Anxiety and How It Affects Mothers

When I first started experiencing anxiety during pregnancy, I felt like I was the only one. It seemed like all the other women I knew were embracing the experience with joy and excitement, while I was drowning in fear and worry. But as I began to open up to my healthcare provider, my therapist, and even other mothers, I realized that I wasn't alone. Anxiety during pregnancy is more common than many of us realize, and knowing that I wasn't the only one dealing with these overwhelming emotions helped me feel less isolated.

Understanding the prevalence of anxiety among pregnant women gave me some much-needed perspective. I learned that pregnancy anxiety can affect anyone, regardless of whether it's their first pregnancy or their fourth, and it's not a reflection of how much you love or want your baby. Anxiety during pregnancy is a real and widespread issue, and acknowledging this fact is an important step toward addressing it.

The Numbers: How Common Is Anxiety During Pregnancy?

When I first started researching anxiety during pregnancy, I was shocked to learn how common it actually is. Studies show that about 1 in 10 pregnant women experience anxiety. That means millions of women worldwide go through the same worries, fears, and stress that I was dealing with. And yet, it's a topic that often feels overlooked or minimized in conversations about pregnancy.

I remember feeling relieved when my doctor explained that anxiety during pregnancy wasn't something to be ashamed of. It wasn't a sign that I was failing as a mother-to-be, nor did it mean I was doing something wrong. My anxiety was simply a natural response to the massive changes—both physical and emotional—that were happening in my life.

But just because anxiety is common doesn't mean it should be ignored. Left untreated, pregnancy-related anxiety can have a real impact on both the mother and the baby. That's why it's so important to recognize the signs early and seek out support and strategies for managing it.

The Emotional Toll of Anxiety on Mothers

For me, one of the hardest parts of dealing with anxiety during pregnancy was the emotional toll it took on me. I wanted to enjoy my pregnancy, to feel the excitement and joy that so many people talked about. But instead, I often felt disconnected from those positive emotions. It was like my anxiety built a wall between me and the happiness I was supposed to feel.

The constant worry about my baby's health, about labor, and about my ability to be a good mother consumed so much of my mental and emotional energy. There were days when I felt completely drained—both physically and emotionally—because I had spent so much time worrying. It's exhausting to be in a constant state of fear, and over time, that exhaustion started to wear me down.

I also struggled with feelings of guilt and shame. I felt guilty for not enjoying my pregnancy as much as I thought I should. I questioned whether my anxiety would affect my baby and whether I was doing enough to protect them. I was ashamed of the fact that, instead of feeling joyful, I often felt terrified.

These emotions compounded the anxiety I was already feeling. It wasn't just the fear and worry that weighed on me—it was the guilt and shame that came along with it. But as I learned more about the prevalence of anxiety during pregnancy, I started to let go of those feelings of guilt. I realized that I wasn't alone, and that anxiety didn't make me a bad mother—it made me human.

How Anxiety Affects Mothers Physically

One of the things I wasn't prepared for was how anxiety would affect me physically. I had always thought of anxiety as a mental or emotional issue, but during pregnancy, it manifested in my body in ways I didn't expect.

The most obvious symptom was sleep disruption. As my anxiety worsened, I found it harder and harder to fall asleep at night. My mind would race with worries, and even when I was physically exhausted, I couldn't quiet my thoughts enough to rest. I would wake up in the middle of the night, heart pounding, and spend hours lying awake, consumed by fears about the pregnancy or the future. This lack of sleep only made my anxiety worse, creating a vicious cycle that was hard to break.

Beyond the sleep issues, my anxiety also caused other physical symptoms. I experienced headaches, muscle tension (especially in my neck and shoulders), and digestive issues. I would often feel nauseous, which was frustrating because it made it harder to distinguish between typical pregnancy symptoms and the physical effects of anxiety. There were times when my stomach was in knots, and I wasn't sure if it was due to morning sickness or stress.

The tension in my body became unbearable at times. My shoulders felt like they were constantly hunched up to my ears, and my back ached from the strain of carrying around all that anxiety. My therapist later explained that this was my body's way of responding to stress. The constant state of alert that anxiety puts you in causes your muscles to tighten, your heart rate to increase, and your body to prepare for "fight or flight"—even when there's no real danger.

Recognizing that these physical symptoms were a result of my anxiety helped me feel less frustrated. It made me realize that my body wasn't betraying me—it was just reacting to the mental and emotional stress I was under. This understanding allowed me to take more intentional steps toward managing both the mental and physical aspects of my anxiety.

The Impact on Relationships

Anxiety during pregnancy didn't just affect me—it also had an impact on my relationships with the people around me, particularly my partner. I was fortunate to have a supportive husband who was there for me every step of the way, but there were times when my anxiety made it hard for us to connect.

I found myself withdrawing from him, not because I didn't want his support, but because I felt like my anxiety was a burden. I didn't want to constantly talk about my worries, and I was afraid that if I opened up too much, he might become overwhelmed or frustrated. This led to moments of isolation where I felt like I was going through the pregnancy alone, even though he was right beside me.

There were also moments when my anxiety caused tension between us. He would try to reassure me that everything was going to be okay, but in the height of my anxiety, I couldn't always accept that reassurance. I would push back, asking endless "what if" questions, and it sometimes led to frustration on both sides. He wanted to help, but my anxiety made it hard for me to feel comforted.

What helped us get through these moments was open communication. I eventually learned to express what I was feeling without expecting him to fix it. I told him that sometimes, I just needed him to listen, to be there with me in the anxiety, even if there were no easy answers. He, in turn, learned to offer support without trying to "solve" my anxiety. This approach helped us strengthen our relationship during a time that could have easily driven us apart.

The Long-Term Impact of Untreated Anxiety

As I began to manage my anxiety more effectively, I learned about the potential long-term impact of untreated anxiety during pregnancy. While occasional worry is normal, chronic anxiety can have lasting effects on both the mother and the baby if it goes untreated.

One of the risks of untreated anxiety is that it can lead to depression, either during pregnancy (known as antenatal depression) or after the baby is born (postpartum depression). For me, the fear of slipping into depression was real, especially since I was already struggling with the emotional and physical toll of anxiety. I knew that if I didn't take steps to manage my anxiety, it could affect my ability to bond with my baby and care for myself in the postpartum period.

There's also evidence that untreated anxiety during pregnancy can lead to complications like preterm birth, low birth weight, or developmental issues in the baby. Learning about these risks was sobering, but it also motivated me to take my mental health seriously. I realized that by addressing my anxiety, I wasn't just taking care of myself—I was taking care of my baby too.

The Importance of Early Intervention

What became clear to me as I went through my pregnancy was the importance of early intervention. The sooner I acknowledged my anxiety and started seeking help, the sooner I was able to regain a sense of control over my mental health.

For me, early intervention meant talking to my doctor as soon as I recognized the signs of anxiety. It meant reaching out to a therapist who specialized in pregnancy-related mental health and learning strategies to manage my stress. It also meant building a support system of friends and family who understood what I was going through and were there to listen and offer reassurance.

By addressing my anxiety early, I was able to prevent it from escalating into something more serious. I learned that while anxiety during pregnancy is common, it doesn't have to define your experience. With the right support and tools, it's possible to manage anxiety and still find joy and peace in the journey to motherhood.

Chapter 5: How I Overcame Anxiety: Treatment Options That Worked for Me

During my pregnancy, the weight of anxiety often felt like too much to bear. It wasn't just the physical discomfort or the constant worries about the future; it was the overwhelming sense of dread that accompanied me throughout the day. At times, I feared that this anxiety would consume me entirely. But through a combination of specific treatments and approaches, I was able to regain control and find peace. Here, I'll share the methods that helped me, in the hope that they can guide you on your journey as well.

Cognitive Behavioral Therapy (CBT): Changing My Thinking Patterns

One of the most pivotal parts of my recovery was Cognitive Behavioral Therapy (CBT). I remember sitting in my therapist's office, my heart racing as I described the constant worries I had—whether my baby would be healthy, whether I could handle the responsibility of being a mother, and the endless "what ifs" that consumed my thoughts. My therapist introduced me to CBT, and it changed everything.

CBT helped me recognize that many of my thoughts were distorted by anxiety. Every time I felt a pang of fear, I would automatically assume the worst: that something terrible would happen to my baby, or that I wasn't capable of being a good mother. Through CBT, I learned how to challenge those thoughts. Instead of spiraling into worst-case scenarios, I began to ask myself, "Is this really true?" and "What's the evidence for this fear?"

For example, if I had a thought like, "What if something goes wrong with the baby?" I learned to replace it with a more balanced thought like, "I am doing everything I can to ensure a healthy pregnancy, and I have a good support system in place."

Guided Self-Help: Taking Control of My Own Recovery

Even though CBT sessions were incredibly helpful, I realized that I needed more than just therapy appointments to manage my anxiety. So, I started exploring guided self-help techniques. I found a workbook recommended by my therapist that focused on managing pregnancy anxiety, and I began dedicating time each day to work through the exercises.

What helped the most was writing down my fears and then reframing them. It was therapeutic to see my thoughts on paper—it made them feel less overwhelming. I'd list out all the things that were bothering me, and then I would challenge each one with a realistic, calming response.

For instance, when I worried about not having enough resources to care for my baby, I would remind myself of all the support I had—my family, friends, and even community resources. This exercise helped me regain perspective, and over time, I found myself feeling more in control.

Mindfulness and Relaxation: Finding Peace in the Present Moment

As part of my healing process, I knew I had to find a way to calm my mind. Anxiety always pulls you into the future—into the "what ifs" and worst-case scenarios. So, I turned to **mindfulness**. At first, it felt impossible to sit still and focus on my breath when my thoughts were racing, but with practice, I found it to be one of the most effective tools for calming my anxiety.

I started each morning with a simple mindfulness practice. I'd sit in a quiet corner of my home, close my eyes, and focus on my breath. I didn't try to stop the anxious thoughts, but instead, I observed them without judgment. This was hard at first because my instinct was always to panic over the thoughts. But over time, I learned that by simply acknowledging the thoughts without letting them control me, they began to lose their power.

I also incorporated deep breathing exercises. Whenever I felt an anxiety attack coming on, I'd stop whatever I was doing and focus on slow, deep breaths—counting to four on the inhale and four on the exhale. This simple exercise became my go-to method for stopping anxiety in its tracks. It reminded me that I had control over my body, even when my mind felt out of control.

Physical Activity: Moving My Body to Calm My Mind

Staying active during my pregnancy wasn't just about keeping my body healthy—it was about keeping my mind healthy, too. I found that gentle exercise, like walking and prenatal yoga, made a huge difference in managing my anxiety. There were days when I felt too overwhelmed to even get out of bed, but on the days I did go for a walk or do a simple yoga routine, I noticed an immediate lift in my mood.

One particular experience stands out. I was about six months pregnant, and I had been feeling particularly anxious about labor. That day, I decided to go for a walk along the beach. As I walked, I focused on the sound of the waves and the feeling of the breeze on my skin. Slowly, I felt the anxiety melting away, replaced by a sense of calm. It was a reminder that moving my body helped release the tension that was building up from my anxiety.

Exercise became an essential part of my routine, not just for my physical health but for my mental well-being. I realized that even small movements—like stretching or walking—could make a big difference in how I felt.

Medication: A Difficult but Necessary Decision

When I first discussed the idea of medication with my doctor, I was hesitant. I didn't want to rely on medication to manage my anxiety, especially during pregnancy. But as my anxiety worsened, I realized that I needed to explore all options to ensure both my and my baby's well-being.

With my doctor's guidance, I started taking a low dose of an SSRI (Selective Serotonin Reuptake Inhibitor), a type of medication commonly prescribed for anxiety. We carefully weighed the benefits and risks, and I felt reassured by the fact that it was a well-researched treatment with minimal risks to the baby.

The medication wasn't a magic fix, but it gave me the extra support I needed to manage the overwhelming feelings. I noticed that my panic attacks became less frequent, and I was able to focus more on preparing for motherhood rather than being consumed by fear. It wasn't an easy decision, but it was the right one for me.

Acupuncture and Massage: Finding Holistic Relief

As my due date approached, I also sought out more holistic treatments to manage my anxiety. I had always been curious about acupuncture, and after reading about its benefits for stress relief during pregnancy, I decided to give it a try. I was surprised by how much it helped. Each session left me feeling deeply relaxed, as though the tension had been physically lifted from my body.

In addition, I treated myself to regular prenatal massages. These massages weren't just a luxury—they were a necessary part of my anxiety management plan. During each session, I felt the tightness in my muscles release, and I would leave with a renewed sense of calm. These treatments became a way for me to nurture both my body and mind during a time when anxiety often felt all-consuming.

Finding What Works for You

Looking back, it was a combination of approaches that helped me overcome pregnancy anxiety. No single method was a magic cure. Instead, it was about finding the right balance between therapy, self-care, physical activity, and (when necessary) medication. What worked for me might not work for everyone, but the most important lesson I learned was this: It's okay to ask for help.

Whether you're managing your anxiety through therapy, mindfulness, or medication, remember that you're doing the best you can for both yourself and your baby. The journey to overcoming anxiety is not a straight path, but with the right support and tools, you can find your calm amidst the chaos.

Chapter 6: Practical Techniques for Managing Anxiety in Pregnancy

Managing anxiety during pregnancy isn't something that happens overnight. For me, it required daily attention, small changes, and conscious decisions to prioritize my mental well-being. I didn't just wake up one day with all the answers—each step I took built on the previous one, and over time, I found myself better equipped to handle the challenges of pregnancy anxiety.

In this chapter, I'll share the practical techniques I used that made a significant difference. These aren't abstract concepts, but real, tangible strategies that helped me stay grounded and calm during some of the most anxious moments of my pregnancy. My hope is that these techniques will provide you with practical tools to apply in your own journey, helping you find peace and reassurance as you prepare to welcome your baby.

Building a Support System: Leaning on Family and Friends

During my pregnancy, one of the most important things I did was build a strong support system. I realized early on that I couldn't go through this journey alone—nor did I have to. I reached out to family and friends, sharing my fears and anxieties with them. At first, I felt hesitant. I worried they wouldn't understand or that they might think I wasn't excited about the baby. But once I opened up, I discovered that people were much more understanding than I expected.

My husband became my rock. He was there on the days when my anxiety felt like it was swallowing me whole. I remember one night in particular when I was overwhelmed with fear about labor. My mind was racing, imagining all the things that could go wrong. Instead of bottling it up, I told him how I was feeling. He listened, reassured me, and reminded me that I wasn't alone. That conversation, simple as it was, helped release the tension I was holding onto.

Beyond my immediate family, I leaned on a close circle of friends. They checked in regularly, offering encouragement and support. One of my friends, who had gone through a difficult pregnancy herself, shared her own experience with anxiety. Hearing that I wasn't the only one struggling helped me feel less isolated.

Finding Your Tribe

In addition to friends and family, I sought out other expectant mothers who were going through the same emotional rollercoaster. I joined an online support group for pregnant women dealing with anxiety. Being able to share my thoughts in a safe, non-judgmental space with others who understood what I was going through was incredibly empowering. The group became a place where I could vent, ask questions, and even offer support to others, which gave me a sense of control.

If you're feeling overwhelmed, don't hesitate to reach out to your partner, friends, family, or even online communities. You might be surprised at how much relief comes from simply sharing your experiences and realizing that you're not alone.

Daily Self-Care: Prioritizing My Mental and Physical Health

One of the hardest lessons I learned during pregnancy was that I needed to prioritize my own self-care. I had always been someone who put others first, but pregnancy taught me that I couldn't pour from an empty cup. The more I ignored my own needs, the worse my anxiety became. So, I made a commitment to myself: I would dedicate time each day to taking care of both my mind and body.

Some days, self-care meant doing something physical, like going for a walk or practicing prenatal yoga. Other days, it was more about mental self-care, like sitting in a quiet space, reading a book, or taking a long, warm bath to relax my muscles and calm my mind.

What made the biggest difference, though, was consistency. I made sure that every day, I did something just for me—no matter how small. Even if it was only for 10 or 15 minutes, that time became sacred. It was a reminder that my well-being mattered, and by taking care of myself, I was also taking care of my baby.

Journaling: Releasing My Fears on Paper

Journaling became one of the most effective tools for managing my anxiety. Whenever I felt overwhelmed, I would sit down with my notebook and write out everything that was on my mind. I didn't filter my thoughts or worry about whether what I was writing made sense. I just let the words flow.

One entry that stands out to me was from a particularly anxious day when I was terrified about labor. My mind was swirling with fears, and I felt like I couldn't catch my breath. So, I wrote down every single fear: "What if I can't handle the pain? What if something goes wrong? What if I'm not strong enough?"

After pouring all those thoughts onto paper, I felt lighter. Seeing my fears written out in front of me made them seem less all-consuming. They were just thoughts, not reality. Journaling helped me process my emotions in a way that felt safe and productive. It gave me space to acknowledge my anxiety without letting it take over.

If you're struggling with anxious thoughts, I highly recommend keeping a journal. It doesn't have to be anything fancy—just a place where you can be honest with yourself about what's going on in your mind. Over time, you may find that journaling helps you understand your triggers and gives you clarity on how to manage them.

Physical Activity: Moving My Body, Calming My Mind

As I mentioned earlier, staying active during pregnancy was one of the most powerful ways I managed my anxiety. But it wasn't about pushing myself to the limit—it was about finding gentle, mindful ways to move my body that also soothed my mind.

Every morning, I would take a short walk around my neighborhood. I lived near a park, and there was something about being surrounded by nature that made me feel grounded. The fresh air, the sound of the wind in the trees, and the rhythmic movement of my feet all worked together to calm the storm inside me. It wasn't just about the physical benefits—though I appreciated how walking helped ease the physical discomforts of pregnancy—it was about the mental clarity that came with it.

On the days when I felt too tired to walk, I would do some gentle stretching or prenatal yoga. I remember one day in my third trimester when I was feeling particularly anxious about labor. I rolled out my yoga mat and followed a simple stretching routine. By the end, I felt more relaxed and less consumed by fear.

Movement helped me reconnect with my body, reminding me that I was strong and capable, even when anxiety told me otherwise.

Sleep: Prioritizing Rest and Recharging My Mind

Sleep was another area where I had to make a conscious effort. Like many pregnant women, I struggled with insomnia, especially in the third trimester. I would lie awake at night, my mind racing with worries. But I knew that without enough sleep, my anxiety would only worsen.

So, I developed a nighttime routine that helped me wind down and prepare for sleep. It included:

- Turning off screens an hour before bed to reduce stimulation.
- Listening to calming music or a guided meditation to quiet my mind.

- Drinking a cup of herbal tea (approved by my doctor) to relax my body.
- Practicing deep breathing to help me fall asleep.

These small changes made a big difference. By prioritizing rest, I was able to recharge both mentally and physically, making it easier to manage my anxiety during the day.

Nutrition: Fueling My Body for a Clear Mind

I also learned that what I put into my body had a direct impact on my anxiety levels. Early in my pregnancy, I noticed that when I ate too much sugar or processed foods, my anxiety would spike. I'd feel jittery and on edge, which only fed my anxious thoughts.

So, I made an effort to eat more whole, nourishing foods—fruits, vegetables, whole grains, and lean proteins. I also stayed hydrated, making sure I drank plenty of water throughout the day. These small changes helped stabilize my energy levels and keep my mind clearer. I wasn't perfect, of course, but I found that when I treated my body with kindness, it responded in kind, helping me stay calmer and more balanced.

Finding Your Own Path

The practical techniques I used during pregnancy weren't a one-size-fits-all solution. What worked for me might look different for you, and that's okay. The key is to find what feels right for you—whether that's building a support system, journaling, practicing mindfulness, staying active, or prioritizing rest and nutrition.

It's important to remember that managing anxiety is an ongoing process. There will be good days and hard days, but each small step you take will bring you closer to a place of peace. You have the strength to navigate this journey, and by taking care of yourself, you're also taking care of your baby.

Chapter 7: How Anxiety Affects Your Baby and What You Can Do About It

One of the most challenging aspects of dealing with anxiety during pregnancy was the constant worry about how it might affect my baby. I was caught in a vicious cycle: the more I worried about my anxiety, the more anxious I became. I asked myself countless times, "Will my anxiety harm my baby? What if all this stress is too much for them?" These thoughts haunted me throughout my pregnancy, but as I learned more and sought advice from professionals, I found ways to manage those fears and protect my mental health—and ultimately, my baby's well-being.

In this chapter, I want to share what I learned about the connection between maternal anxiety and the baby, and most importantly, the steps I took to keep both myself and my baby healthy and thriving.

My Worries About the Impact of Anxiety

As my pregnancy progressed and the anxiety intensified, I began to obsess over whether my constant worrying and stress would negatively affect my baby. I read articles about how maternal stress could lead to low birth weight, premature birth, or developmental issues, and this information made me even more anxious. It was a never-ending cycle: the more I worried about the impact on my baby, the more anxious I became, which only reinforced my fears.

But something shifted when I finally decided to speak to my doctor about it. She reassured me that while anxiety is common during pregnancy, the key is recognizing when it becomes overwhelming and taking proactive steps to manage it. What mattered most was finding a balance and making sure that I wasn't letting anxiety consume me.

What I Learned: The Effects of Anxiety on Babies

Through my conversations with healthcare providers and my own research, I learned that moderate anxiety, especially when it's managed, is unlikely to cause any harm to the baby. However, chronic, untreated anxiety can have effects, and understanding those helped me feel more empowered to manage my mental health. Here's what I learned:

- Stress Hormones: When we experience prolonged anxiety, our bodies release stress hormones like cortisol. During pregnancy, these hormones can cross the placenta, exposing the baby to higher levels of stress. This was something I was deeply concerned about, but my doctor reassured me that occasional anxiety wouldn't harm the baby. It was the chronic, unaddressed stress that could potentially pose risks.

- Potential Risks: Research suggests that prolonged, severe anxiety during pregnancy might be associated with a higher risk of preterm birth, low birth weight, or developmental delays. But it's important to note that these risks are typically linked to extreme, untreated anxiety. For most women—myself included—the key is managing anxiety before it becomes chronic and seeking help when needed.

- Emotional Bonding: I also worried about whether my anxiety would affect my ability to bond with my baby. Would I struggle to connect with them emotionally because I spent so much time worrying? Thankfully, this fear didn't come true. What I learned was that by managing my anxiety, I could create a healthier mental space for myself, which helped me bond with my baby during pregnancy.

Taking Action: What I Did to Protect My Baby

Once I understood the potential effects of anxiety on my baby, I became even more determined to manage it. I knew that the best way to protect my baby was to take care of myself first. Here are the steps I took to ensure that my baby was safe and healthy, even as I navigated my own mental health challenges:

1. Prioritizing Self-Care

As I mentioned earlier, self-care became an essential part of my daily routine. But this wasn't just about feeling good—it was about creating a calm environment for my baby. I knew that when I was taking care of myself—whether that meant eating well, getting enough sleep, or practicing mindfulness—I was also taking care of my baby. I made self-care a priority not only for me but for them.

There were days when I felt guilty for taking time to rest or step away from responsibilities, but I reminded myself that reducing my stress levels was one of the most important things I could do for my baby's health.

2. Practicing Relaxation Techniques

One of the techniques that had the most direct impact on my anxiety—and, by extension, my baby—was practicing deep relaxation exercises. Whenever I felt my anxiety creeping in, I would pause, close my eyes, and focus on my breathing. I used simple techniques like **deep belly breathing** (inhaling deeply through the nose, holding for a few seconds, and exhaling slowly through the mouth) to calm both my mind and body.

Over time, these practices helped me lower my stress levels. I would often imagine my baby during these exercises, visualizing the calm environment I wanted to create for them. It gave me a sense of control, knowing that by calming myself, I was creating a safer, more peaceful environment for my baby.

3. Limiting Exposure to Stressful Information

One of the hardest things I had to do during pregnancy was limit my exposure to information that triggered my anxiety. At the height of my anxiety, I found myself constantly researching potential risks—reading stories of difficult pregnancies or medical complications. While I thought I was being prepared, I was actually feeding my anxiety.

So, I made a conscious decision to cut back on reading articles or engaging with social media posts that heightened my fears. I focused instead on trusted sources of information, like my healthcare provider and evidence-based websites. This shift made a huge difference in my mental state. I was still informed, but I wasn't overwhelmed by negative stories that fed into my anxiety.

4. Seeking Professional Support

There were moments when my anxiety felt too much to handle on my own. During those times, I sought help from professionals who specialized in prenatal mental health. My therapist became a lifeline, helping me work through my fears and teaching me coping strategies that made a tangible difference in my day-to-day life.

If you're struggling with anxiety during pregnancy, I can't stress enough the importance of seeking help. Whether it's through therapy, talking to your doctor, or finding a support group, having professional guidance made all the difference for me. It wasn't just about reducing my anxiety—it was about ensuring that I was doing everything I could to create a healthy environment for my baby.

5. Communicating with My Baby

One of the more surprising techniques I used to manage my anxiety was talking to my baby. I know it might sound strange, but whenever I felt overwhelmed, I would place my hands on my belly and talk to my baby. I would tell them that everything was going to be okay and that I was doing everything I could to take care of them.

These moments of connection helped me focus on the bond I was building with my baby, rather than getting lost in my fears. It was a reminder that I wasn't alone—my baby and I were in this together, and by calming myself, I was helping them too.

The Power of Managing Anxiety

By taking these steps, I felt a sense of empowerment. I realized that while anxiety is normal during pregnancy, it doesn't have to take control. I was able to create a calm, nurturing environment for my baby, even when I was dealing with my own mental health struggles. The most important lesson I learned was that by managing my anxiety, I was not only taking care of myself but also protecting my baby.

Every step you take toward managing your anxiety is a step toward giving your baby the best possible start in life. Don't be afraid to prioritize your mental health—you and your baby deserve it.

Chapter 8: Managing Fear of Labor and Delivery (Tokophobia)

One of the most intense sources of anxiety I experienced during pregnancy was the fear of labor and delivery. It was a fear that crept in quietly at first, but as my due date approached, it became louder and harder to ignore. I couldn't shake the "what ifs" running through my mind: What if the pain is unbearable? What if something goes wrong? What if I'm not strong enough to make it through labor? This fear—often referred to as tokophobia, the fear of childbirth—became one of the biggest challenges I had to overcome.

In this chapter, I'll share how I faced my fear of labor head-on, the techniques I used to manage those feelings, and how I ultimately found the strength to trust my body and the process of childbirth.

My Fear of the Unknown

Like many first-time mothers, the fear of the unknown was a huge source of my anxiety. I had heard so many stories about labor, and while some of them were positive, others painted a terrifying picture of pain, complications, and things spiraling out of control. My mind became fixated on these worst-case scenarios, and I found myself dreading the day I would go into labor.

As my due date grew closer, the fear started to take over. I remember waking up in the middle of the night, my heart racing, as I imagined myself in the delivery room, feeling completely unprepared and powerless. I began to question my own strength: Could I handle the pain? What if I panicked? What if I wasn't as strong as I hoped?

This fear made it hard to enjoy the final weeks of my pregnancy. Instead of focusing on the excitement of meeting my baby, I was consumed by thoughts of the pain and uncertainty of childbirth.

Taking Control of My Fear

I knew I couldn't let this fear paralyze me. As much as I wanted to avoid thinking about labor, I realized that ignoring my fear wasn't going to make it go away. So, I decided to take control by learning as much as I could and preparing myself both mentally and physically. Here are the steps I took that made a real difference in managing my tokophobia.

1. Educating Myself About Childbirth

One of the first things I did to manage my fear was educate myself about the process of childbirth. I signed up for a childbirth class where I learned about the different stages of labor, pain management options, and what to expect during delivery. At first, the information was overwhelming. I felt nervous just hearing about contractions and the pushing phase. But the more I learned, the more empowered I felt.

Understanding what my body would be going through gave me a sense of control. I learned about natural pain relief methods, such as breathing exercises and relaxation techniques, and I also learned about medical interventions, like epidurals, that would be available if I needed them. Having this knowledge helped me feel less like a passive participant and more like an active part of the process.

I also made a birth plan, which included my preferences for pain management, who I wanted in the room with me, and any specific requests for the delivery. While I knew that labor doesn't always go according to plan, having a general outline of my wishes gave me a sense of agency.

2. Reframing My Thoughts About Pain

One of the hardest things for me to accept was the idea of pain. I was terrified that the pain of labor would be more than I could handle. But through my childbirth classes and conversations with my healthcare provider, I learned that pain during labor isn't just something to fear—it's a natural part of the process, signaling that my body is doing exactly what it needs to do to bring my baby into the world.

I started to reframe my thoughts about labor pain. Instead of seeing it as something unbearable, I began to view it as something purposeful. Each contraction was a step closer to meeting my baby. This shift in mindset was difficult at first, but it made a big difference. I reminded myself that millions of women have gone through labor, and while it's not easy, it's something I was built to handle.

One phrase that stuck with me was, "The pain has a purpose." I repeated this to myself whenever I felt my anxiety about labor creeping in. It helped me focus on the end goal—a healthy baby—and reminded me that the pain wasn't permanent.

3. Practicing Relaxation and Breathing Techniques

In addition to educating myself about labor, I practiced **relaxation and breathing techniques** that would help me stay calm during contractions. I found these techniques incredibly helpful, not just during labor but also in the weeks leading up to my due date when my anxiety about childbirth was at its peak.

I practiced **deep breathing exercises** every day, focusing on slow, controlled breaths. One technique that I found particularly helpful was **rhythmic breathing**, where I would inhale for a count of four, hold for a count of four, and exhale for a count of four. This method helped calm my racing heart and kept me focused on the present moment.

I also tried **visualization exercises**. I would close my eyes and imagine myself in a peaceful place—somewhere that made me feel safe and calm, like a quiet beach. I visualized myself breathing through contractions, staying calm, and feeling in control. These visualization exercises helped me mentally rehearse for labor, making it feel less like an unknown, terrifying event and more like something I could handle.

4. Talking About My Fears with My Doctor

Another step that helped ease my anxiety about labor was talking openly with my doctor. I shared my fears about childbirth—everything from the pain to the possibility of complications. My doctor was incredibly understanding and reassured me that my fears were normal. We discussed pain relief options, and she walked me through what would happen in case of any complications, like the need for a C-section.

Having these conversations gave me a sense of relief. I realized that I didn't have to go through labor alone. I had a team of professionals who would be there to support me every step of the way. My doctor also encouraged me to trust my body and the process. She reminded me that my body was designed for this, and that I had the strength to get through it.

5. Building a Supportive Birth Team

Having the right people around me during labor was another key part of managing my fear. I knew I wanted my husband by my side—his calm presence was a huge source of comfort for me. We practiced breathing exercises together and talked about how he could support me during labor. Just knowing that he would be there, holding my hand, made me feel less afraid.

I also made sure to communicate my needs to my healthcare team. I let them know that I was feeling anxious about labor and asked for their reassurance and guidance throughout the process. I wanted to feel like I had a supportive team around me, and by being open about my fears, I was able to build that sense of trust and connection with my birth team.

6. Letting Go of Perfection

Perhaps the biggest lesson I learned in managing my fear of labor was letting go of the need for perfection. I realized that childbirth, like pregnancy, is unpredictable. While I could make a birth plan and prepare myself mentally, I couldn't control every aspect of labor. And that was okay.

I let go of the idea that labor had to go exactly as I imagined. Instead, I focused on staying flexible and trusting that whatever happened, I would have the support I needed. This mindset shift helped alleviate a lot of my anxiety because it took the pressure off trying to control every detail.

When the day finally came, and I went into labor, I wasn't without fear. But I felt more prepared than I had in the months leading up to it. I used my breathing techniques, leaned on my support team, and trusted that my body was capable. It wasn't an easy experience, but it was a powerful one. And in the end, it brought me my beautiful baby, which made every moment worth it.

Finding Strength in Vulnerability

Labor is one of the most intense experiences a woman can go through, and it's normal to feel afraid. But I learned that the strength to face that fear comes from acknowledging it, preparing for it, and trusting yourself. There's power in vulnerability—in admitting that you're scared but choosing to move forward anyway.

If you're struggling with fear of labor, know that you're not alone. It's okay to be afraid, but it's also okay to trust that you're stronger than you think. By educating yourself, practicing relaxation techniques, and building a supportive birth team, you can face labor with confidence and grace. You've already come so far on this journey—and you have everything you need within you to handle whatever comes next.

Chapter 9: Finding Your Calm: Daily Habits for Long-Term Peace

As I moved through my pregnancy, I learned that managing anxiety wasn't just about finding quick fixes—it was about developing daily habits that helped me stay grounded and calm, even during the most stressful moments. These habits became my anchors, providing stability when everything around me felt overwhelming. They weren't elaborate or complicated, but they made all the difference in helping me maintain my mental health during pregnancy and beyond.

In this chapter, I'll share the daily habits that worked for me and how they can help you cultivate a sense of calm and peace as you navigate your pregnancy. These aren't just tools to use in the moment—they're habits that can help you build long-term resilience and mental well-being, even after your baby arrives.

1. Starting the Day with Intention: Morning Mindfulness

One of the most important habits I developed during my pregnancy was starting each day with mindfulness. In the past, I had always jumped right into the day, checking my phone or rushing to get things done. But during pregnancy, I realized that how I started my day set the tone for everything that followed. If I started my morning in a rush, I was more likely to feel anxious and overwhelmed later on.

So, I made a conscious decision to begin each morning with a few minutes of mindfulness. It didn't have to be anything fancy—sometimes it was just sitting quietly with my cup of tea, focusing on my breath, or taking a few deep breaths before getting out of bed. This small act of mindfulness helped me start the day with a sense of calm and focus.

I often found myself placing my hands on my belly and talking to my baby during these quiet moments. I'd say things like, "Today is going to be a good day," or "We're in this together." It was a way to ground myself and connect with my baby before the chaos of the day began.

If you're struggling with anxiety, I encourage you to try starting your day with intention. It doesn't have to be complicated—just a few minutes of quiet reflection can make a big difference. Whether it's focusing on your breath, journaling, or simply sitting in silence, finding a calm moment at the start of your day can set a positive tone for everything that follows.

2. Moving My Body: Gentle Exercise for Mental Clarity

Physical activity became another cornerstone of my daily routine during pregnancy. I discovered that when I moved my body, my mind followed. Even on days when I felt tired or anxious, going for a short walk or doing a few gentle stretches helped clear my head and reduce the tension I was holding onto.

For me, walking became a form of moving meditation. I'd head outside, focus on the rhythm of my steps, and let the movement help me release any anxiety I was carrying. Some days, I'd listen to calming music or a podcast, but other times, I'd just walk in silence, paying attention to the sights and sounds around me. The fresh air and gentle movement worked wonders for both my body and my mind.

Prenatal yoga was another favorite of mine. I found that the gentle stretches and focused breathing helped ease the physical discomforts of pregnancy while calming my racing thoughts. I wasn't an expert by any means, but I loved how yoga helped me feel more connected to my body and more in control of my emotions.

You don't need to engage in strenuous exercise to reap the mental health benefits. Even something as simple as a 10-minute walk or a few stretches can help release tension and clear your mind. The key is consistency—making physical activity a regular part of your routine can help reduce anxiety and improve your overall sense of well-being.

3. Staying Present: Letting Go of "What Ifs"

During my pregnancy, I often found myself caught up in "what if" thinking. What if something goes wrong? What if I'm not ready? What if I can't handle motherhood? These thoughts would spiral in my mind, creating a constant undercurrent of anxiety. I knew that to find peace, I needed to break free from this cycle of worry.

One of the most effective techniques I learned was staying present. Whenever I felt myself getting lost in "what if" thinking, I'd bring my attention back to the present moment. I'd ask myself, "What's happening right now?" and focus on what was directly in front of me. It might be something as simple as the sound of my breath, the feeling of the chair beneath me, or the sight of my baby's ultrasound picture on the table.

Staying present helped me recognize that most of my fears were about the future—things that hadn't happened and might never happen. By focusing on the present, I was able to let go of the worries that were out of my control and find peace in the here and now.

If you're prone to "what if" thinking, try practicing mindfulness or grounding techniques to bring yourself back to the present. Even something as simple as naming five things you can see or feel around you can help you break free from anxious thoughts and return to the moment.

4. Journaling: Reflecting on My Journey

Journaling became one of my most powerful tools for managing anxiety during pregnancy. There was something incredibly therapeutic about putting my thoughts on paper. It allowed me to release the worries that were swirling in my head and see them more objectively.

Some days, I'd write about my fears—everything that was making me anxious. Other days, I'd focus on the positives, like the things I was excited about or grateful for. I found that both approaches were helpful in different ways. Writing about my fears helped me process and release them, while writing about my gratitude helped me shift my focus to the good things in my life.

One of the most impactful exercises I did was writing letters to my baby. I'd write about how excited I was to meet them, how much I already loved them, and how I was doing everything I could to take care of them. These letters became a way to strengthen the bond between me and my baby, even before they were born.

If you haven't tried journaling yet, I highly recommend giving it a go. You don't need to be a writer or have a fancy journal. Just grab a notebook and write whatever comes to mind. It's a simple, effective way to process your emotions and gain clarity on what's really important.

5. Setting Boundaries: Protecting My Peace

As I navigated my pregnancy, I realized that not every conversation or piece of advice was helpful for my mental health. There were times when well-meaning friends or family members would share horror stories about labor or offer unsolicited advice that only heightened my anxiety. I had to learn to set boundaries to protect my peace.

At first, this was difficult for me—I didn't want to offend anyone or seem ungrateful for their support. But I realized that my mental health needed to come first. I started gently steering conversations away from topics that made me anxious. If someone began sharing a negative story, I'd say something like, "I appreciate your concern, but I'm trying to stay focused on positive thoughts right now."

Setting boundaries also extended to the information I consumed. I limited my exposure to stressful news stories and avoided reading too much online about rare pregnancy complications. Instead, I focused on positive, evidence-based resources and surrounded myself with people who were supportive and uplifting.

If you find that certain conversations or pieces of information trigger your anxiety, don't be afraid to set boundaries. It's okay to protect your peace by limiting your exposure to negativity. Your mental health—and your baby's well-being—are worth it.

6. Ending the Day with Gratitude

Just as I started my day with mindfulness, I ended each day with gratitude. Before bed, I'd take a few moments to reflect on the day and think about the things I was grateful for. Some days, it was as simple as feeling grateful for my health or the fact that I had made it through another day of pregnancy. Other days, I'd feel gratitude for the little kicks I felt from my baby or the support I received from my husband.

Ending the day with gratitude helped shift my focus from what was worrying me to what was going well. It reminded me that even on the hardest days, there were always things to be thankful for.

You can try incorporating a gratitude practice into your bedtime routine. It doesn't have to be elaborate—just a few moments of reflection on what you're grateful for can help you end the day on a positive note and sleep more peacefully.

Creating Your Own Routine

The daily habits that helped me find calm during pregnancy were simple but effective. They weren't about making drastic changes or adding more to my plate—they were about making intentional choices to prioritize my mental and physical health. Over time, these habits became second nature, and they helped me feel more grounded, less anxious, and more prepared for the journey ahead.

As you navigate your own pregnancy, I encourage you to find the habits that work for you. Whether it's mindfulness, movement, journaling, or setting boundaries, the key is consistency. By incorporating these practices into your daily routine, you can cultivate long-term peace and resilience, not just during pregnancy but well into motherhood.

Conclusion

Embracing the Journey and Finding Your Calm

Looking back at my pregnancy journey, I see it as a time of immense growth, not just physically but mentally and emotionally. It wasn't always easy—there were days when the anxiety felt overwhelming, when the fear of the unknown clouded my excitement for the future. But through it all, I learned valuable lessons about resilience, self-compassion, and the power of taking things one day at a time.

The most important thing I learned was this: anxiety is real, but it doesn't define you. There were moments when I felt consumed by my fears, but each time, I found a way to rise above them—whether through therapy, mindfulness, self-care, or the support of those around me. Pregnancy brought many challenges, but it also brought opportunities to grow stronger and more confident, not just as a mother but as a person.

Your Journey to Calm

If you're reading this and struggling with anxiety during your pregnancy, I want you to know that you're not alone. The fear, the worry, the overwhelming thoughts—these are things many of us face, and it's okay to feel uncertain or afraid. What matters is how you move through those feelings and take steps to care for yourself.

Remember that every small step counts. Whether it's taking a few moments of mindfulness in the morning, going for a walk to clear your mind, or reaching out to a loved one for support—these actions all contribute to a stronger, more peaceful state of mind. The journey to calm isn't about being perfect; it's about being patient with yourself, trusting the process, and knowing that you are doing your best for both yourself and your baby.

A New Chapter Begins

As I moved beyond pregnancy and into motherhood, I found that many of the habits and techniques I developed stayed with me. The mindfulness, the self-care, the support systems—they weren't just tools for pregnancy; they became part of my daily life as a new mother. And that's the beauty of this journey: the skills you learn to manage anxiety during pregnancy will serve you long after your baby is born.

Motherhood comes with its own set of challenges, but having gone through the experience of managing anxiety during pregnancy, I felt more prepared to face those challenges. I had built a toolkit of strategies that helped me stay calm and grounded, even when things felt chaotic. And I know that you, too, can carry these lessons forward with you into the next phase of your life.

You Are Stronger Than You Think

One of the greatest realizations I had during this journey was that I was much stronger than I ever gave myself credit for. There were times when I doubted my ability to cope with anxiety, to handle labor, or to be a good mother. But with each challenge I faced, I discovered a well of inner strength that I didn't know existed.

You have that strength within you, too. Even on the days when anxiety feels like too much, remember that you have already made it this far. You are stronger, braver, and more capable than you may realize. Trust yourself, trust your body, and trust the journey.

Final Thoughts

As I finish writing this book, I am filled with gratitude—for the lessons I learned, for the support I received, and for the beautiful life that came from this experience. My hope is that by sharing my story, I can offer you comfort, reassurance, and practical tools to help you navigate your own journey with anxiety.

Remember, anxiety is a part of the journey, but it doesn't have to control it. You have the power to manage your fears, to find peace in the midst of uncertainty, and to embrace this incredible experience of bringing new life into the world.

Together, we can find calm—one step, one breath, and one day at a time.

About the Author

Bonaventure Paul is an accomplished writer and father of two who has gained firsthand insight into the challenges women face during pregnancy through his own experiences supporting his wife. His personal connection to the pregnancy journey made many of the emotional and physical aspects highly relatable, fostering a deep empathy for the experiences of expecting mothers. Bonaventure's writing is driven by a commitment to provide thoughtful guidance and support to families navigating similar challenges.

This book is based on an interview Bonaventure conducted with a nursing mother, who candidly shared her struggles with pregnancy-related anxiety and how she overcame them. Through this real-life account, Bonaventure brings the reader into a personal and inspiring story of resilience, offering practical insights for managing anxiety during pregnancy. His goal is to share this powerful experience to help others on their journey to parenthood.

Bonaventure Consults

Disclaimer

This book is based on a real-life experience shared during an interview with a woman who overcame anxiety during pregnancy. The content provided is intended for educational purposes and is meant to offer guidance and insight into managing pregnancy-related anxiety. However, it is important to note that the information in this book should not be used as a substitute for professional medical advice, diagnosis, or treatment.

Every pregnancy is unique, and while the techniques and strategies shared here may be helpful, they are not one-size-fits-all solutions. If you are experiencing anxiety, depression, or any other mental or physical health concerns during pregnancy, we strongly recommend consulting with a physician, therapist, or other qualified healthcare professionals who specialize in pregnancy-related issues. Always seek the advice of your healthcare provider with any questions you may have regarding your pregnancy or mental health.

The author and publisher of this book are not responsible for any adverse effects resulting from the use or application of the information contained within. The reader assumes full responsibility for their actions and decisions based on the content provided in this guide

Acknowledgement

Thank you so much for purchasing 'Calm Pregnancy'. Your decision to invest in this book means the world to me, and I truly hope it offers you comfort, guidance, and the reassurance you need during your pregnancy journey. It has been a privilege to share this story and these insights with you, and I'm grateful for the opportunity to support you in this special chapter of your life.

Your feedback is incredibly valuable. If this book has helped you in any way, I would be honored if you could take a moment to leave a honest review. Your thoughts will not only help me improve but will also guide other expectant mothers who may be looking for encouragement and support.

Thank you again for trusting me to be a part of your journey, and I wish you peace, strength, and joy as you move forward toward motherhood.

Printed in Great Britain
by Amazon